Dopamine Detox to Address Depression and Anxiety

A Practical Guide to treating the most "common cold" of mental health in the nation

Gerald Smith

© **Copyright 2021 - All rights reserved.**

The content contained within this book may not be reproduced, duplicated or transmitted without direct written permission from the author or the publisher.

Under no circumstances will any blame or legal responsibility be held against the publisher, or author, for any damages, reparation, or monetary loss due to the information contained within this book, either directly or indirectly.

Legal Notice:

This book is copyright protected. It is only for personal use. You cannot amend, distribute, sell, use, quote or paraphrase any part, or the content within this book, without the consent of the author or publisher.

Disclaimer Notice:

Please note the information contained within this document is for educational and entertainment purposes only. All effort has been executed to present accurate, up to date, reliable, complete information. No warranties of any kind are declared or implied. Readers acknowledge that the author is not engaged in the rendering of legal, financial, medical or professional advice. The content within this book has been derived from various sources. Please consult a licensed professional before attempting any techniques outlined in this book.

By reading this document, the reader agrees that under no circumstances is the author responsible for any losses, direct or indirect, that are incurred as a result of the use of the information contained within this document, including, but not limited to, errors, omissions, or inaccuracies.

Table of Contents

Table of Contents 4

Chapter 1: The Pursuit of Pleasure 7

   Human History of Dopamine Addiction...........................7

      The difference between pain and discomfort 14

      If discomfort was a drug, you'd take it 16

Chapter 2: Dopamine...23

   What is Dopamine? 23

      Signs of dopamine deficiency 29

      Diseases caused by dopamine deficiency 30

      Dopamine and mental health 31

      Dopamine provides pleasure 31

      Addiction and dopamine..32

      Addiction treatment...33

   How to Plan a Dopamine Detox.....................................34

   How to Reduce Dopamine Resistance 38

   Dopamine Tolerance 43

      What causes an excess of dopamine? 46

      Does dopamine excess cause anxiety?.......................47

Drugs containing dopamine are used in the treatment of which diseases?... 47

Dopamine and serotonin 47

Dopamine addiction or dopamine dependency? 48

Drugs for the Determined 48

Chapter 3: Balancing Comfort and Discomfort 55

What is Anxiety? 55

Trying to combat anxiety 56

Happiness and discomfort 57

Dopamine for fear... 58

Dealing with discomfort 59

The Home Called Comfort Zone 60

Comfort zone = golden cage? 61

Fear leads to self-sabotage 62

Are you in the comfort zone out of fear of loss? 63

Meditation for anxiety relief..................................... 66

Best meditation types for anxiety 67

Best meditation types for depression 68

Keeping a meditation journal 69

Why Spirituality is Important.......................................70

The Depression-Discomfort Defense............................. 71

Dangers of avoiding 72

> Perception or reality 73
>
> Horror 73
>
> Obscurity 74
>
> References 77

Chapter 1: The Pursuit of Pleasure

Human History of Dopamine Addiction

Addiction is the continued use of a substance despite negative effects on health and daily life. Many factors can be and often are underlying during the development of an addiction. Some of these factors can be fundamental things such as personal or family problems, not being able to get away from daily struggles, and/or having been bullied. People from all kinds of backgrounds can become addicted and it is not exclusive to a specific social-economic class. Furthermore, addictions can occur unexpectedly, even if we are vigilant about our behavior and our surroundings. We mustn't be so hard on ourselves for our weaknesses but work to overcome them, instead.

When you get into the grip of addiction, your view of the world may narrow, and you can only focus on the substance or activity you are addicted to. Everything other than that, like friends, family, and work, loses its importance.

The only thing that makes the addicted person feel good is the choice of the substance to which they are addicted because they are seriously lacking natural dopamine production either due to the addiction or some previously occurring illness. Dopamine is necessary for one to feel pleasure, but the most intense forms of pleasure aren't just elicited by a high circulating level of dopamine. No, intense pleasure is elicited by a large *change* in circulating dopamine, not simply high concentrations of the stuff. High basal dopamine levels generally cause a decrease in its overall effects, especially when the high circulating levels are being chronically induced by an addictive substance. When the dopamine regulation mechanism does not work correctly, a person can seek other ways to be happy. In many situations, this can lead to long-term use of addictive substances and substance abuse.

"Pain is the oldest medical problem," said Marcia Meldrum, an associate researcher at the University of California, Los Angeles (Collier, 2018). She and other scientists agree on the fact that while pain might be as old as time, it has been poorly understood.

Pain teaches us more than a lot of other feelings do. Said practically, pain teaches us what to fear. Said more esoterically, pain provides the motivational foundation for aversive stimuli in all organisms, including humans. Said bluntly, pain hurts. If we can pay attention to this sensation, pain offers a learning experience on its own. For example, dull throbbing pain is often transmitted by projections from neurons whose axons are unmyelinated, resulting in a lower speed of propagation and generally indicating some form of internal discomfort or damage. If you don't understand this jargon that's okay; these concepts will be further elucidated throughout the course of this book.

While it might help us learn a lot about life, pain is undesirable. We fear it, we do not want to feel it, and the feeling of it gives us anxiety, sadness, and in some situations, even depression. Depending on how bad it is, pain can either be a minor inconvenience or flip your life upside down. In the history of humanity, we have always had to deal with pain and if we know one thing, it is that we will always have to deal with it in the future, as well as dealing with the problems our "treatments" may create.

Thankfully, through the advent of scientific discovery and drug design, there are ways to ease and even treat pain, but is easing your pain a good thing? Did you know that doctors used to think that pain was good for us? They thought the lack of pain would result in a longer time frame for healing. While this thought was disproven, more recent studies suggest that opioid usage slows wound healing, especially in seniors. In a study published by Temple University in 2017, researchers found that subjects who did not take opioids healed faster than the subjects who received opioids of 10mgs or more a day (Unterwald et al., 2017).

When we look at how mankind has dealt with pain over history, we see that neither doctors nor the public considered pain without clear pathology to be serious up until the 1900s. It was often believed that people, who were not injured or dying from noticeable diseases, were either crazy, lying about their pain or that they were trying to abuse drugs (Goldberg, 2017).

Drug abuse related to pain problems is not new. It started around 3,400 B.C. when opium was invented with red poppies. Up until the 1800s, when organized governments were starting to regulate medical ingredients, opium was still used to treat pain. However, opium was only used for serious, fatal pain and nothing else. Everyone else who wanted opium due to pain was not taken seriously. The 1800s was the time ether and chloroform were starting to be used in surgeries as anesthesia. While some doctors felt a little strange about operating on unconscious individuals, they now had more control, more time, and an increased ability to treat medical problems. It is not hard to believe that the patients preferred the anesthetics, even when the possible side effects were made clear.

Sometime in the early 1900s, stronger medications began being distributed and used as pain medications. Two of these medications were morphine and heroin. The seriousness of both drugs being addictive was very conflicting for many doctors. They wanted to help their patients, but did not want to subject them to the grip of addiction. This was also around the time chronic pain was becoming more accepted by doctors and more drugs were prescribed to people who did not have cancer, obvious injuries, or surgeries before the prescription. Now, people who doctors believed to be in pain for whatever reason, could get access to painkillers. Prior to the availability of pain-relieving drugs, patients who suffered from pain would often turn to neurosurgery or psychotherapy to ease their pain. Techniques which proved to unreliable when it comes to their results. Some people would have great results from the limited treatment options, whereas others would continue to complain about their pain.

It might be easy to tell that someone is in pain if the pain is extreme and they are crying or screaming, but how about the less extreme cases of pain? We cannot tell if someone is in pain by simply just looking at them. "The only way to know if someone is in pain, is to ask them," Meldrum said (Collier, 2018). Unfortunately, there is not an exact way to measure how much pain a person is in and people, especially people who are addicted to drugs, can lie. This makes the topics of pain, painkillers, and addiction very controversial. Is pain all in our heads? Can we control it with our brains? How realistic is it to believe that not thinking about pain improves it? Well, Meldrum suggests that pain is in our heads to an extent. We know we are in pain; this causes us to have feelings of anxiety and the anxiety helps add to the pain (Collier, 2018). The anxiety you experience from being in pain, makes you hurt even more, like the well-known fact that when a child falls, they may not react negatively until you do. You are not supposed to make a noise or react until they do because even if the child is not hurt, your reaction might give them anxiety about the situation and convince their brains that they, in fact, are in pain and make them cry. Pain and anxiety go hand in hand.

When you realize that you are in pain, your brain reinforces the idea repeatedly. This is called anxiety. The best thing to do when you are in pain is to attempt to redirect your attention away from the pain. A task much easier theory than in practice. As a result, the field of medicine has always turned to drugs when it comes to pain so maybe "not thinking about it" is not as easy as we might think. We will investigate how we can use our heads to ease pain in the next chapter of the book. For now, let's continue talking about the history of mankind's fatal obsession with not being in pain.

At the end of World War II, veterans came back to the US, rightfully expecting healthcare services. Opioid prescriptions and usage went up significantly due to the veterans in chronic pain who needed treatment. This started the pain epidemic of the 1940s. While the public was confused about the pain treatment options offered to the vets, they were supportive of the people who fought for them in the war. Around the 1950s, the number of veterans who needed chronic pain and disability treatment had skyrocketed up to 3 million (Bernard et al.,2018). Pharmaceutical companies started to realize that the opioids were selling like hotcakes and there was no end in sight. The needs of veterans are important, but we did not understand pain or painkillers back then. This made it hard to control dosage and even addictions.

However, in 1968, the Gate Control Theory of Pain was published. The theory helped shine a much-needed light on the psychological, spiritual, and physiological effects of pain in humans. This showed that pain, whether from war or not, can cause a lot of mental harm and suffering for a person (Mendell, 2014). These effects were seriously overlooked by doctors and scientists all over the globe for the last 4000 years so it was a big deal, to say the least. Finally beginning to accept the effects of culturally learned stoicism on human psychology and how it can cause feelings of anxiety and depression, the funding for pain research and treatment options increased all around the world.

Around the 1970s, the war on drugs started and made substances like marijuana, LSD, and heroin harder to come by. This caused a direct increase of prescribed opioids, creating a demand higher than the supply. Pharmaceutical companies arose to the occasion and got new drugs on the market to satisfy the demand. At first, when the usage of painkillers grew from only acute pain patients to chronic pain patients, opioids were recommended to only be taken in a hospital environment and be supplemented with behavioral and psychological care. However, this was just a recommendation and not a rule, and opioid usage largely shifted to routine at home patient self-administration.

Finally, in 1977, The American Pain Society was founded to conduct better research on acute and chronic pain. By the 90s, society had begun to gather controversy as it received huge funding from pharmaceutical companies. During these times, many flawed theories about opioid usage were being acknowledged by The American Pain Society. Between 1990 and 1995, the number of opioid prescriptions went up by 2 to 3 million after Purdue Pharma advertised their new painkillers as non-addictive. This was false information, and the company was fined a large sum of money for "knowingly disseminating false information" back in 2007. Unfortunately, it was too late to stop the effects of the drug on the people who had used it before the lawsuit, and the drug was responsible for fueling the usage of opioids for chronic conditions. You cannot help but wonder how so many people are in this much pain. Opioids are supposed to be for extreme chronic or acute pain, after all. Non-opioid painkillers such as paracetamol have been on the market for a very long time and can treat pain without being addictive. One of the things that make opioids addicting is that they tend to come with a side effect of a high or a feeling of intense euphoria. This does not happen with other non-addictive painkillers. So while the intended use of prescription painkillers is to stop or dull pain, what people are addicted to is the feeling of euphoria rather than the lack of pain. Substances such as endorphins, dopamine, serotonin, GABA, and epinephrine come to the fore in research on smoking, alcohol, and substance abuse.

Between drugs, an increased consumer-product accessibility, and the availability of the internet, it may be easy to get overstimulated sometimes for some people. For these people, the pleasure which they experience from big events gets smaller and smaller because their dopamine receptors are used and abused. This occurs when a high circulating level of dopamine is maintained or induced through repeated use of addictive substances. In the short-term, minutes to hours, this can cause reduced sensitivity to the substance. While long term activation, hours to days, can lead to cells removing some of their external dopamine binding sites all together. It is recommended for surviving opioid addicts to do a dopamine detox to help them along with their treatment. We'll get into how to do a dopamine detox and investigate ways we can promote dopamine production other than synthetic drugs, in the next chapter.

Throughout history, humans have always found a way to get high. Opium, cannabis, mushrooms, minerals, bugs, and many other things that we can find in nature have gotten us nice and happy when ingested but with the rise of technology and science, some of these natural things have morphed into very dangerous drugs. The way we look at pain is simple; we don't want it. The opposite is happiness, which we always want. But what if the presence of a little amount of pain was helpful for your overall happiness in life? Maybe not pain but what if discomfort could actually help you thrive?

The difference between pain and discomfort

Pain and discomfort are words that are often used in the same context meaning the same thing on different levels. But, they can and often do mean different things. The simplest way to distinguish the two is to think of pain as a feeling that does not improve by pushing through whereas discomfort gets better over time when pushed through. Take for example yin yoga. During yin yoga, the yogi gets in a pose where they remain for a couple of minutes. At first, the muscles hurt and want to be relieved but after 30 seconds or so, the muscles start to relax and flex, providing a deeper pose and a better exercise. The "hurt" our muscles feel during this time could be labeled as discomfort as it got easier to tolerate as time went on. Now, imagine that while you are getting in the pose, you accidentally bruised one of your hamstrings. This could be labeled as pain because what you need after this "hurt" is not to push through but rather to rest and relax the muscle until it is healed. Although discomfort does not always mean pain, small amounts of pain can also be described as discomfort. To put it simply, while pain can be one of many of the contributors to discomfort, not every discomfort can be labeled as pain. It is like how all thumbs are fingers but not all fingers are thumbs.

When pain is extreme or intense, it cannot be avoided. It needs attention and more often than not, rest. Discomfort is more on the annoying side; it is there, you can feel it, and you don't like it but you are able to tolerate it. It might even help you step out of your comfort zone. Discomfort and growth have more of a connection than we might realize.

In the modern world, we often treat pain and discomfort the same way. We want it gone! However, as we discussed earlier because they are not the same thing, we cannot use the same treatments when getting rid of both. If you are in pain because you broke your leg, getting a cast and taking painkillers will help you no longer be in pain but if you were to try and "walk it off", you would end up hurting yourself more. In situations of discomfort, though, if your leg hurts because your muscles are stiff, stretching and walking it off would help you. The next time you use those muscles, you will be more comfortable doing so. The path and result of not wanting to be in pain is usually just that, not being in pain. But the path to not being in discomfort usually crosses through more discomfort and anxiety before you reach your goal which will leave you at a better place than you started. It is easy to grasp the concept of discomfort producing growth, but we all know that actually stepping out of your comfort zone can be very hard for some people.

John C. Maxwell once said, "Growth demands a temporary surrender of security," and it makes a lot of sense (Rogers, 2015). Nobody ever learns or becomes anything until they step out of their comfort zone. Discomfort is not like pain when you look at it from this point of view. Both pain and discomfort are an inconvenience to us while we are living through them but while pain might continue and hurt us in the long run, the discomfort usually helps us learn from the situation. Bodybuilders don't go to the gym every day for 2 years and do the same exercises with the same weights. They must push themselves forward. What they experience is discomfort. So maybe, we can learn from yogis and bodybuilders to see discomfort as an opportunity to achieve excellence. Not surprisingly, doing activities that will push you to and through your limit has the same chemical effect on our bodies as the euphoria humans feel from prescription painkillers. This chemical effect is called the release of dopamine, the pleasure neurotransmitter.

You may or may not have heard of dopamine, but you love it and that is a fact. Neurotransmitters are little messengers your brain sends to your body to do or feel different things. Dopamine neurotransmitters help us feel pleasure. They help us to be more focused and find life a little more interesting. We will get into how dopamine is made in the next chapter. But in the next section of this chapter, we will discuss why feeling discomfort might end up making you a happier person in the long run.

If discomfort was a drug, you'd take it

Unless you have a fetish for it, none of us like to be uncomfortable or in pain. We have spent decades and billions of dollars trying to make life as comfortable for ourselves as possible. However, the benefits of discomfort really do outweigh the misfortunes of it.

When we learn how to walk, we fall and then get right back up to try again. Sometimes we might scrape a knee, or hurt ourselves, but even when we are infants, we know that practice makes perfect. Eventually, we learn to walk without falling and even start running! Do you think a baby who doesn't know that they can walk yet, knows that they can run? Even the fastest runners in the world had to learn how to walk first. So, now, think about a scenario where when the fastest runner in the world was a baby, their parents were so worried about them hurting themselves that they didn't let them learn how to walk. The world would never know their name. Your anxiety can sometimes act as the parents in this scenario and keep you from living your life to its fullest potential.

Our comfort zones start developing when we are just babies. We learn to play and push boundaries so that we can develop a unique set of skills and a one-of-a-kind personality. We often think of our adolescent years fondly because as children, we produce a lot of dopamine. I mean, when you are a kid, you have fewer responsibilities; people are literally in charge of taking care of you, your food is put in front of you, and you get to do and learn new things quite regularly. Our brain is fascinated by the new information we gather and it rewards us with the pleasure messenger. Over time, the regularity of us learning new things decreases and we end up not having as much dopamine in our lives as we used to as things become routine. Think about the first time you saw your favorite movie and then think about the last time you've seen it. Is it still just as exciting? Or does the pleasure you get from watching it have to do with the nostalgia of it and not the actual movie? Plenty of people seem to find themselves stuck in the past. They simply refer to those times as "the good old days" but is it the goodness of the old days or the pleasure we felt when things were new and exciting to us?

We simultaneously don't want things to change but also want things to get better. Time and time again people will set goals they never even begin to accomplish. You will most certainly hear people make new year's resolutions about losing weight or getting in shape because they no longer feel comfortable in their own bodies but very few of them will eat right and exercise. It is easy to want to look and feel good but to get up and workout every few days, cutting out junk food, carbonated drinks, alcohol, and carbs can be extremely hard in a world where transportation is personalized, and grocery stores are full of sugary treats. Once you give up your goal because it is too hard to reach, you are less likely to try again. But what if you succeed? How would that feel? Would you feel happy or sad that you started? If you saw that what you are doing is giving you results, wouldn't you keep going? It would be a motivator for you. Your brain produces plenty of reward dopamine when you accomplish things you set out to do.

Looking at opioid addiction from a dopamine point of view makes things look a little sadder but clearer. Opioids make people feel happy because the drug helps produce dopamine. When a person is hungry, they eat, and the hunger is gone. When they are tired, they sleep and they wake up energetic. However, when a person is sad and they cry, they become sadder. There is no direct way to be happy so when someone is starved of happiness, they might turn to drugs to make them feel a slight sense of pleasure. Drug addicts often suffer from mental or physical health problems that dragged them into the addiction in the first place. Depression alone can be held responsible for many addictions. The story is similar regarding anxiety. Our lives are stressful. We must balance work, friends, family, hygiene, social activities, and more things all at once. On the other hand, these stressful situations can also become routine and put us on autopilot for weeks at a time.

The modern human is not challenged enough. Our brains love to be challenged. We love learning new things, overcoming problems, getting through tough situations, and especially being recognized and praised for the good we have done. The only problem is that we are also all programmed to remain at the status quo. There is a "way" to do everything, which is what we learn from a young age. You are born, you go to school, then college, you get a job with benefits for your future, you get married, you have kids, you retire and then you die. This is the circle of life. There are plenty of routines throughout this life that have already been laid out in front of you. It is easy to get caught up in the big picture and not pay attention to things that might lead you to experience depression, anxiety, or even burnout. With life being so routine, we feel less challenged because we feel like we are doing what is expected of us. Our brains end up eating up the small amount of dopamine we make due to small events and there is not much left to spare. Drugs can seem like the easy way out of feeling like yourself again. The "self" that was happy once, like when you were a kid. But what if you did something else that made you feel like you did when you were a kid? What if you challenged yourself? It could be the simplest thing. It is like a little bet with yourself. Science says that pushing your own boundaries and slowly getting out of your comfort zone can drastically improve a person's life.

The key to your best self is discipline and a little bit of discomfort. Growing our comfort zones is vital to becoming a happier person. Think of the most spoiled child you know; can you already tell that they are going to be horrible and entitled people? This is because people whose comfort zones are underdeveloped, often do not know how to handle discomfort and make it everyone else but their own responsibility to get out of that discomfort. It makes sense to think that the less discomfort you were subjected to as a child, the less you know how to deal with the situation.

Unsurprisingly, the only way to grow out of your comfort zone is to be uncomfortable for a little while. It is important to remember that seeking comfort aggressively and constantly might negatively affect your long-term happiness. Like a knife, unless it is being sharpened, your dopamine levels can become famished, making you seek things to make you feel happy again. It is good to have a stable, not dangerous life, but are you still finding ways to better yourself? When was the last time you felt proud of yourself? The more you create and experience, the more your brain creates new and different pathways. These pathways help you improve your memory and get your creative juices going.

I am not trying to make pain and suffering sound like good things in this book. There are discomforts that we cannot treat and situations no humans should live through, of course, but I am talking about the parts of our lives we can strategically alter to benefit us in the long run. The old saying "no pain, no gain" almost has the correct idea. Without pushing your limits, those limits will not grow. For example, studies have shown that taking cold showers triggers something called a cold shock protein that helps heal diseases, especially brain-related ones. Cold shock proteins protect the neuron connections, providing our brains with both short and long-term help. Taking cold showers, or getting into ice baths might be uncomfortable but doing so helps boost the production of CSP. The discomfort of being submerged in or under cold water might sound terrible at first but by doing it often, you get used to it. Therefore, after a while, you can take your cold showers without being too distressed and still reap the benefits of the cold water.

Being in unfamiliar situations triggers a very specific part of your brain that gets the dopamine going. This part of your brain is only ever active if you are experiencing new things. When we experience pain, dopamine levels plummet and this makes us understand that pain equals unhappiness. While this is true, a lot of artists throughout history have sought out pain and suffering to create great works of art, in the pursuit of happiness.

Movies like *Rocky, Captain America, Yes Man,* and many more are based on the principle of discomfort triggering discipline. Men who normally would be considered unfit, train hard to become the best around, or a man who usually never says no practices saying yes often and it improves his life in a major way. We all know a successful someone who nobody believed in at first. It might even be you. If you want to be a generally happy person, you must subject yourself to discomfort when;

- You can do it step by step

There is no need to rush any growth process if you want to do it right. Set your growth goal. It could be anything from making dinner every day of the week to building a rocket ship in your backyard (not recommended). Now break that goal into smaller goals you can accomplish in the short term. Like if it is the dinner goal, make today's goal to do your grocery shopping and put the items away. If it is the rocketship, maybe start with doing research on the regulations. Achieving your goal in small steps might actually make you cherish it a lot more in the end while still getting small releases of dopamine in the meantime thanks to your short-term goals.

- You feel safe

While it is great to get out of your comfort zone and push yourself to do new, different things, you must make sure that you are not pushing yourself too far out of your comfort zone to a place you might never want to go again. When you don't test the waters and jump in, you might feel overwhelmed and conclude that the goal is too hard to achieve. This may even make you not want to try new things again. When you decide to do something new, make sure to have a clear understanding of what might happen. Reassure yourself that even if you experience feelings of anxiety, you will come out stronger on the other side. If the anxiety feels too much to handle, it might be time to put on the breaks for a little bit while you take a breather. It is okay to take a moment to yourself and get back into things when you are refocused. You've got this.

- The result has great benefits

You are the master of your own life. When you think of your life, you should be the captain and the pilot behind the wheel. Think of what you want your life to be like. Unless you are super lucky or have done great amounts of work on yourself, there is no way you can get where you want your life to go by being the same exact person you are now. The result of your growth will be your dream life. You might hate working out, but if you have a supermodel body in your dream life, you must start heading to the gym more often. If you want to become the best chef in town, you've got to start trying out new recipes.

There are countless ways to use discomfort to push yourself to have a happier life. The sky's the limit. Producing dopamine is an important part of our lives. We seek dopamine without even knowing what it is or that we need it. We simply consider happiness to come from the events that happen around us, not necessarily that it comes from within us. This is why plenty of people turn to drugs, to feel a sense of pseudo happiness. Could we learn how to live without dopamine?

Chapter 2: Dopamine

In this chapter of the book, we will learn more about dopamine, where it comes from, how it is distributed around our bodies, and what kind of behavioral and lifestyle factors help boost the production of nature's happy chemical messenger.

What is Dopamine?

Despite what some may believe, happiness is indeed within us. The human brain is an incredible thing. It can make you feel everything or if it chooses to, nothing. All of our physical and emotional feelings are made in our heads and distributed through our bodies.

Questions such as what dopamine does and how it even does it, have been controversial in the neuroscience industry for decades. More than 110,000 studies have been released about dopamine but it remains to be a controversial topic among scientists (Powledge, 1999). Dopamine is a neurotransmitter. This neurotransmitter helps us feel all of our feelings and helps us control and regulate our movement. It even helps with our attention span and learning. It also allows not only to see possible rewards but also to take action to move towards them. One of the things it is responsible for is sending the signals between our nerve cells.

Chemical messengers in the brain are called neurotransmitters. These messengers are then attached to molecules called receptors. The job of these receptors is to move the neurotransmitter that is carrying the signal from one cell to the other. Very few neurons make dopamine and not every transmitter is made in the same part of the brain either. Dopamine gets produced in three separate parts of the brain: the substantial nigra area, the ventral tegmental area, and the arcuate nucleus of the hypothalamus. All of these brain areas might be tiny but they are solely responsible for our dopamine needs.

- The substantia nigra area: Dopamine produced from the substantia nigra area helps to initiate movements and speech.

- The ventral tegmental area aka VTA: The functions of dopamine produced in this part of the brain are less well defined and are the main source of controversy among neuroscientists. Dopamine that is produced in the VTA does not directly help people move or do things. What it does is that it sends dopamine to the brain when we expect a reward. It could be the simplest thing like your favorite food or a good classic song from your teen years. Not all neurons in the VTA make dopamine. Many studies suggest that the sudden appearance of unwanted or harmful stimuli, such as pain, causes the activation of certain neurons in the ventral tegmental area.

Finally, the pyriform complex of the olfactory bulb is responsible for providing humans with a sense of smell. In the mesolimbic pathway, dopamine is released in pleasurable situations. It causes arousal and motivates behavior for pleasurable activity or pursuit. It binds to dopaminergic receptors located in the nucleus accumbens and prefrontal cortex. Here, it binds to dopaminergic receptors and transmits signals. Thus, it takes part in the following roles:

- situation assessment and analysis function

- engine control mechanism
- motivation
- behavior reinforcement
- reward mechanism

The functions of dopamine in our body are too many to count. Dopamine is decisive in almost all the functions of the brain and is the main motivator behind our actions and our relationships with other people.

Below are the most basic functions of dopamine:

- Dopamine and mobility

The basal ganglia is responsible for all of our brain-controlled movements. But, if we want our basal ganglia to work without problems, the neighboring neurons have to release a lot of dopamine. If not, the basal ganglia will encounter restrictions and affect our abilities to move. If enough dopamine does not reach the basal ganglia, we may encounter restrictions in our ability to move or disordered movements.

Excessive production of dopamine can cause the body some problems as well. For example, too much dopamine can cause you to make unnecessary movements. It is a little-known fact that the main reason for the uncontrollable repetitive movements known as 'tics' is the excessive production of dopamine by neurons.

Sometimes the cells that make our dopamine supply die unexpectedly. Surprisingly, scientists still do not know why that happens. Researchers are currently investigating the role genetics play, environmental factors, and the natural aging process in cell death and Parkinson's disease, a disease where one has uncontrollable hand tremors. It can occur in men and women around the age of 60. Some people develop Parkinson's disease early (around the age of 40).

- The effect of dopamine on memory and learning

The prefrontal cortex, which is involved in thinking and memory, is often associated with dopamine. Even minor fluctuations in the amount of dopamine in the prefrontal cortex can directly and significantly affect memory. In addition to the learning processes, dopamine also has an effect on which and how information is stored.

Dopamine helps us remember happy memories that spark joy better than the not-so-happy ones. You can also get your prefrontal cortex to produce some dopamine when you participate in a favorite activity.

- Effect of dopamine on attention and focus

Dopamine works by responding to the optic nerves, which allow you to focus on a certain subject or thing. Lack of dopamine and low dopamine concentration in the prefrontal cortex can cause you to have trouble paying attention and focusing.

- How dopamine affects perception

Dopamine determines how we perceive our experiences and events. Dopamine, which is released when we are pleasant, causes us to want to do this pleasant activity again in the future. For example, dopamine is the reason why we want to eat our favorite foods again and get pleasure from sexual intercourse. In short, dopamine allows us to take pleasure from our actions, just like the hormone serotonin.

- Dopamine, stress, and excitement

Dopamine is also produced in high amounts when we encounter situations and events that excite us or cause sudden stress.

Therefore, excessive dopamine secretion can bring about stress, anxiety, and tension in the person.

- Effect of dopamine on mood

Dopamine, a chemical that releases feelings of pleasure and is decisive on our mood. Why we enjoy some events and hate others can be explained by our internal production and release of dopamine from the brain areas mentioned previously. Dopamine is often called the "happy" molecule and a lack of it can trigger depression.

- Dopamine addiction

Drugs like cocaine and amphetamines target neurotransmitter proteins that regulate the release of dopamine in the brain. Alcohol, cocaine, and other drugs slow down the communication between neurons by mimicking GABA neurotransmitters; At the same time, they create a desire to take these substances again.

When we say that these compounds mimic GABA, we are more specifically saying that their chemical structure allows them to act in a similar fashion as GABA does in the brain. But when we compare the structure of alcohol and GABA, we can see that alcohol is less than half the size of GABA, so how exactly is that similar? Well, GABA acts in the brain by binding to a receptor on the surface of neurons, acting like a key fitting into a lock and making it less likely for that neuron to fire. Usually, the large difference in size prevents much alcohol from binding to GABA receptors, especially at low concentrations. This is when people feel "tipsy". At high concentrations of alcohol, the size difference doesn't matter much because for every one molecule of GABA there are multiple molecules of alcohol. As a result, there is a much higher likelihood that alcohol will bind to the receptor and cause an inhibitory response. This can lead to serious and noticeable inhibition of the central nervous system, slowing speech and reducing coordination. This is when people feel drunk. Increasing the concentration of alcohol molecules further can lead to a serious deactivation of the central nervous system which will eventually prevent normal functioning necessary for breathing and can lead to death.

Dopamine transporters are responsible for moving dopamine back inside neurons being released. This is a part of neurotransmitter recycling so that the cell doesn't have to make dopamine every time it wants to release it. Cocaine blocks dopamine transporters and leaves dopamine trapped outside the cell. As a result, dopamine binds again and again to the nearby receptors overstimulating the cells. Like other drugs, cocaine concentrates in the reward pathway of the substantia nigra, but also concentrates in parts of the brain controlling voluntary movements like the caudate and putamen of the basal ganglia. This is why cocaine users are fidgety and unable to be still.

Cocaine, alcohol, amphetamines, and most other drugs are small molecules that bind to large receptors and the challenge of understanding how they bind to their receptors has been undertaken by the practice of biochemistry. To describe the way in which they bind their molecules, the "lock and key" model was first described by Emil Fischer in the early 1900's , but more modern science has shown that these receptors usually change shape after binding and are more dynamic. This has led to a modern understanding of receptor binding more like a firm handshake, where each person's hand changes shape to fit the other hand better.

- Effect of dopamine on sleep patterns

Dopamine, which is released more during the day, is produced in lesser amounts late in the evening. Contributing to the natural sleep wake cycle and causing drowsiness near the end of the day. The reason why Parkinson's patients tend to sleep all the time is the insufficient secretion of dopamine. Patients with psychosis, neurosis, and schizophrenia, in whom dopamine is over-produced, also tend to sleep a lot.

- Motivation

In the absence of dopamine, which is released in order to get rewards and achieve good things, we experience a loss of motivation. Therefore, it has important effects on motivation and personal success.

This chemical, which is produced in greater amounts in creative people, enables these people to solve different problems and develop a different perspective on events.

Signs of dopamine deficiency

There are multiple signs of dopamine deficiency, and they will be listed here for your benefit. Keep in mind, this list is not meant to replace the proper diagnosis of a medical professional. The signs of dopamine deficiency are:

- Tremors and loss of balance
- Weight loss or weight gain
- Muscle cramps, spasms, and stiffness
- Eating and swallowing difficulties
- Unfocused and low energy
- Feeling tired and sluggish
- Unexplained sadness

- Moving slower than usual
- Hopelessness, suicidal thoughts, and feelings of guilt
- Hallucinating
- Lack of self-awareness
- Worry and anxiety

Dopamine deficiency can have multiple causes. These causes are often related to mental health disorders. Drug use, an unhealthy diet, and consumption of foods high in sugar and saturated fat can also lead to this deficiency. This is the main reason why obese people are deficient in dopamine. Due to the lack of dopamine, many health problems can develop in us.

Diseases caused by dopamine deficiency

Dopamine deficiency causes multiple disorders, but each disorder is characterized by a slightly different version of the deficiency, either by changing the affected brain region or the type of cell in the brain that is affected. All the following diseases are characterized by some form of dopamine deficiency:

- Social phobia and Psychosis
- Depression
- ADHD
- Insomnia and Anhedonia
- Parkinson's disease

In Parkinson's, the dopamine deficiency is well described by the brain's loss of an ability to produce dopamine due to the death of dopamine producing cells in the Substantia Nigra. Parkinson's disease shows its first symptoms in the form of tremors in the fingers and hands. The disease is further accompanied by symptoms such as excessive sweating, weight loss, and depressed mood.

Lack of dopamine can cause the loss of nerve cells in certain areas of the brain, and for other diseases on this list, the fluctuations in dopamine processing are more subtle.

Dopamine and mental health

In addition to dopamine deficiency, excessive secretion of dopamine can also trigger mental problems. For example, it is known that dopamine is produced excessively in the brains of schizophrenic and bipolar patients. In addition, the person may experience an excessively cheerful mood, high blood pressure, and accelerated heartbeat. The patient may experience results such as hyperactivity, paranoia, stress, restlessness, insomnia, tension, anxiety, and inattention. Dopamine deficiency can lead to mental problems such as depression and social phobia.

Dopamine provides pleasure

Dopamine also affects mood. Dopamine is what drives a lab animal to press a lever repeatedly, for example, to get tasty food. This is why people want to eat another slice of pizza, the taste has a rewarding response from our brains. Reward and reinforcement both help us learn where we can find the important things like food and water so that more can be obtained. Surviving a negative event can also be considered a reward. We experience a lot of pleasure when we accomplish rewarding things. Without dopamine, or with lower amounts of it, you would not be able to enjoy things as simple as eating and drinking as much as you would have with regular dopamine production. This goes for both humans and other animals; less dopamine *generally* results in less pleasure. There is a name for this unpleasant state. It is called anhedonia, or the loss of pleasure.

Addiction and dopamine

Dopamine is a pleasurable chemical that acts on activity and enthusiasm. When the brain creates too much dopamine under the influence of the substance, it stops the production to protect itself. This is why a person feels worse the day after they drink alcohol; one of the hallmarks of hangovers is a dopamine deficiency. The addicted person will tend to increase the dose of the drug they are using to experience the same pleasure they had when they first got a taste of those extra boosts of dopamine.

What drug addiction and Parkinson's disease have in common is insufficient dopamine levels. People who produce smaller amounts of dopamine may be prone to addiction more than those who don't. A specific dopamine receptor and its presence in our brains can be associated with seeking sensations and taking risks. Dopamine is a chemical that affects many things that are important for most everyday behaviors. Most importantly, it affects mental health and enjoyment, increases motivation, and makes the person happy. The use of alcohol, cocaine, stimulants such as nicotine, and other substances like heroin increase dopamine production in some way. This ascent forces people to seek these drugs again and again, even if they are fatally harmful.

Short-term use of chemical drugs also produces the same reward and pleasure for almost all humans. What is okay about that is that things quickly go back to the way they were. However, exposure to drugs can desensitize us to them over time and make us way more tolerant to the drug than we should be. The person now needs even more of the drug in order to get the same positive emotions that once occurred naturally, which is the initial reason to take the drug. Long-term excessive drug or alcohol use hijacks the brain, controlling emotions, motivation, and mood.

In time, these drugs take charge of your dopamine production and replace your receptors. If you don't do the drug that initiated the dopamine boost, you will have very sparse productions of dopamine, running right back to the drug to make you feel alive. Addiction is the source of that person's happiness so, it is definitely not an easy thing for them to stop.

Addiction treatment

The treatment of substance addiction varies according to the characteristics of the addictive substance and individuals. Substance addiction treatment can be done in three ways;

- Normal treatment
- In-patient treatment at a treatment center
- Prevention therapy

The treatment process of substance addiction is possible with intense effort, keeping it under surveillance for 2-6 weeks and following a psychotherapy process. Psychotherapy methods such as cognitive behavioral therapy, group therapy, family therapy, and Bioresonance (Mora therapy) are used in the treatment of this process.

Dopamine function can be restored to its normal state with the help of things like psychotherapy, medications, and other treatments. This may take some time, depending on the duration of use, the degree of use, and the substance of choice. It is always recommended to work with a trained medical addiction specialist, rather than trying to heal alone but there are some things you can do to kick start your healing process. We will get to that in just a little bit.

Safe and effective remediation is possible. Long-term or excessive use of drugs and alcohol can irreversibly alter brain structures and behavior. However, with treatment, the addicted person can learn how to live with brain and behavioral changes. Plenty of recovering addicts live a great life post-addiction thanks to their treatments but unfortunately, addiction cannot be cured completely. The responsibility has to fall back on the patient at one point and it is entirely up to the patient to continue on with their sober life or go back to their addiction, as they can relapse even with one single use of any drug.

How to Plan a Dopamine Detox

Whether it's reckless driving, overeating, or drug addiction, we all have habits that would be considered unhealthy. Unfortunately, the dopamine diet is not the definitive solution, and you may still need some professional treatment, but it can be a good start, especially if you are in the early stages of your habit. It is important to remember that the sooner you start fixing your life, the better.

Experts think that a dopamine detox is a great strategy as long as you don't go overboard with it (MD, 2020). In fact, research shows that in order to deprive yourself of dopamine, you can do very simple things like seeing the dessert tray at a party and walking past. Choosing to avoid desserts is a very effective yet simple way to help yourself detox. The only trick of the dopamine detox is that you are the one responsible for making the right decision. It would be unreasonable to expect there to be no dessert at a dinner party, or to expect the dessert table to run away from you. What must happen is that you have to take responsibility and consciously make the decision to not eat the deserts. This applies to everything you want to do for your detox; you must be the one to follow through. Remind yourself that you've got this and let's get into it.

- **Be decisive!**

  All the decisions you've made so far in your life have brought you here. You have all of the power you need within you. This decision has to begin with you saying, "enough," and taking a step against your dopamine cravings. Decide to be happy in the long run and promise yourself to follow the detox.

- **Set a deadline**

  Having a set time makes things feel more urgent and important. Your well-being is very important, so begin with setting a deadline for how long you are going to do this detox. It could be a month or a year, basically, however long you want it to be. Just remember to stick to the original deadline. If you feel like it would help, start setting smaller goal deadlines before your ultimate one.

- **Write it down**

Keeping a journal of how you feel is often shown as a teen girl thing in movies. However, writing down how you are feeling, what you are doing, and what you are looking forward to has some benefits. It keeps us aware of our mindset, keeps us accountable, helps with motivation, and reduces anxious thoughts along the way.

- **Plan thoroughly**

As mentioned in the previous chapter, forcing yourself too far out of your comfort zone can have catastrophic results. To make sure that you are not overdoing it and therefore giving up soon after, plan your detox thoroughly. Make a list of things you are and are not going to do through your detox and abide by the plan you've made. This list will be your guide. Having a clear guide will help make you stick to your detox plan easier.

- **Involve others**

You are not alone in this. There is always either someone that loves you and will help you get through this or someone who is going through something similar and might be able to offer a supporting hand. Just remember that you are not the only person going through this. Technology and the availability of everything have made us all a little desensitized to dopamine. Involve others in your detox process. Someone you trust will be able to hold you accountable if you slip back into your old habits.

- **Take purposeful action**

Becoming a go-getter is a lot easier than you might think. The secret to it is actually no secret at all: you go and get. Deciding to do something and making a plan for it is wonderful, but only if you actually do them. Leave your phone at home and go out for a walk in nature. No phone, no music, no distractions. Just you and nature. Whatever you do, do the things that will get you to your goal. Set up reminders and alarms as a way of planning your actions.

- **Welcome failure**

    Let's face it, we don't succeed in everything. It might be disappointing to not succeed at first but would be unnatural to accomplish everything we set out for ourselves on the first try. Failing something doesn't have to be a sad situation, instead, you can learn from your mistakes and try your best to not do them again. It is always good to remember that you will only fail until you succeed. Eventually, you will get it right. Just keep going at it with the best attitude even if you fail your detox on your first try.

- **Inspect what you expect**

    Expecting realistic results from your detox is totally vital for this process. If you were 300lbs, you wouldn't expect to be 150lbs just because you went to the gym for 2 days. Spread out your plan and continuously have a conversation with yourself about the outcome of your detox. It is okay to have your expectations shift one way or another depending on how the process is going, however, always be in touch with yourself about what you really expect to come out of this detox.

- **Reward yourself for what you achieve**

    It is extremely important to reward yourself for the small things as well as the big things. If you only expect to be rewarded for the big things, it can be easy to become discouraged. Think about carrying 100lbs up 10 flights of stairs. Would you expect yourself to go all the way up the first time you pick it up? No. You would probably end up taking multiple breaks. Taking these breaks does not mean you're not making progress. It just means you'll get there a little later but safer and less tired. That's why you should reward yourself for every step. The rewards should be things that will make you happy in the short term, without affecting your treatment.

- **Maintain personal integrity**

    You are an adult, in charge of your own life. No one is coming to save you. If you want something, you have to be the one to do it. Having the understanding that no one owes you anything and that life is not always fair is a good thing. It keeps you on your toes. Respect yourself, your future, and your loved one's future enough to actually pull through with your detox. Be honest with everyone, starting with yourself. Keeping your journal and sticking to your plan will definitely help you complete the detox without any problems.

How to Reduce Dopamine Resistance

Now, let's look into some ways you can reduce your dopamine tolerance. Dopamine is the brain's pleasure, motivation, and reward chemical messenger. One can become tolerant to the amount of dopamine they are producing, directly causing them to not feel the effects of dopamine as much as they should or want to. Sometimes, people can then look elsewhere, like to drugs, to find the dopamine they need in order to feel happy. There are ways to naturally raise dopamine levels without the need for opioids even if you feel like you're lacking dopamine highs without them.

Your dopamine detox will include the things below. You don't have to do all of them, though. You can pick and choose the ones you will stick with for the duration of your detox. The more of these things you can add to the list, the better. While they might sound extremely hard for now, you will have the fantastic experience of replenishing your dopamine receptors later on. Keep in mind that your detox can be the turning point of your life. The type of things you can do to detox your dopamine receptors will depend on your individual life and what you usually do when you go seeking dopamine. Do you pick up your phone and go on Instagram, eat three burgers back to back, or reach for the medicine cabinet for a little painkiller activity? Your answer will determine your detox path. Things you can do to detox your dopamine receptors include, but are not limited to:

- Basic self-care!

This is the first step to start raising your regulated dopamine levels. Getting a great night's sleep. Your body rejuvenates when you sleep. This means it fixes the things it can't fix when you are awake. Waking up refreshed and rested will definitely make you feel better and more motivated about life. Make sure to keep activities like showering and brushing your teeth regularly as these will also help you feel more put together and confident. An irregular night's sleep can severely reduce dopamine levels. Therefore, a good sleep and hygiene routine should be followed.

- A balanced diet and increased physical activity!

Maintaining a balanced diet and staying physically active contributes to your overall health and well-being. There are certain foods that increase dopamine sensitivity and should be avoided. It is necessary to stay away from processed foods, junk food, sugar and sweets, and concentrated sources of calories that contain large amounts of brain-destroying dopamine. Consuming too much-saturated fat also reduces dopamine receptor sensitivity. Keep your diet balanced, full of fiber, healthy fats, and carbs. Try an air fryer if you simply cannot live without fried foods. It is life-changing.

- Less time in front of the TV!

Some people can easily become addicted to the time they spend watching television. It is easy entertainment and, when done in the right amounts, it helps promote dopamine production. There is a lot of new content designed to draw the viewer in and keep them watching. Less time watching TV will help your body give your body a chance to reduce your dopamine levels, eventually regulating it enough for you to not be dependent.

- Go on social media less!

Internet usage time should be reduced as well as TV watching time, because internet addiction, which can also be sub-categorized as social media addiction, is an increasingly common problem in the modern world that affects a lot of people, especially the youth. Social media can enrich life by allowing you to connect with old friends and share important moments in one's life, but if not managed properly, it can become a time-consuming addiction that can affect work, relationships, and of course, dopamine levels. Take some time for yourself and remember that what you see on social media is not real anyway. Those people are not as happy as they are pretending to be. You do not need to be in competition with anyone for happiness.

- This means less YouTube as well!

The most popular video streaming website, YouTube is full of entertaining and easily reachable content. It is an entertainment platform with a very addictive potential that can lead to you feeling like you have wasted a lot of time sitting in front of your computer or phone. These types of feelings usually trigger feelings of anxiety and depression. YouTube viewing should be reduced as much as possible while you are doing your detox to focus on yourself.

- Pause the video games for a while!

Video games can sometimes be addictive, depending on what kind of content you play, how you play, and how long you play. The habit of playing video games can be hard to overcome, but getting away from video games for sure will give your brain the break it needs.

- Hydrate, not caffeinate!

Caffeine is a lot of people's first choice of beverage in the morning. Coffee can help you feel more alert and get through the day a little easier. However, drinking too much and for too long can be bad for the health of your brain. Excessive caffeine consumption increases dopamine concentrations in brain synapses. Quitting caffeine cold turkey can be extremely difficult for some people but the benefits heavily outweigh the pleasure. Caffeine is a drug and like any drug, when getting rid of it, you must be prepared for withdrawal symptoms and a drastic drop in your energy levels.

- Carbonated drinks are a no-go!

Although soft drinks seem harmless, they contain a lot of sugar and mess with your brain. They do this by influencing the chemistry of the limbic system. Your limbic system is a part of the brain that is associated with emotional control. Having too much sugar at once and then not having any can lead to a similar behavioral and neurochemical change in the brain as drug addiction. Limiting your carbonated and sugary drink intake is a must during this process.

- NO alcohol!

Alcohol affects the receptor sites of neurotransmitters such as GABA, (gamma-aminobutyric acid, our anti-anxiety neurotransmitter), glutamate (a principle neurotransmitter), and dopamine. Alcohol's activity in the brain's reward center, the dopamine area, boosts the happy, pleasurable feelings that are responsible for a person's desire to drink in the first place. This is why it is important to reduce the intake of booze and focus on your healing.

- NO DRUGS!

This goes without saying but let's say it anyway to have it materialized. Some drugs can be as powerful as boosting your dopamine levels by 12000% above what it is supposed to be. When your dopamine levels get that high, that fast, your receptors end up being all burned up. This causes a person to become addicted to the drug because the only time they can feel happiness is now via a drug. Therefore, absolutely no drugs would be the best way to go during your detox.

- Give the self-pleasure a break!

Sexual pleasure is enjoyable, but too much of a good thing can become a bad thing. Overdoing it with masturbation can lead to a serious case of dopamine addiction, increasing the threshold for satisfaction. This is a key aspect of resetting the dopamine metabolic pathways. Giving yourself a break from masturbation will also help you have a better sexual life in the future. It might be a moot point to mention since masturbation is off the table, but pornography and explicit images cause large amounts of dopamine to be released in the brain. Combined with masturbation, explicit images are some of the most extreme stimuli an individual can encounter, and these are not productive towards the goal of your dopamine detox. So, let's eliminate these two artificial sources of dopamine for the purposes of this detox.

Dopamine Tolerance

As long as the person continues to use the addictive substance, the brain adapts to this situation and gets used to it. To normalize fluctuating dopamine levels, it reduces its own natural production of dopamine and lowers the number of receptors, areas of the brain that dopamine stimulates. Therefore, the addicted person starts to use more drugs to bring the dopamine level to "normal", which we call tolerance.

Drugs that act on the dopamine reward system have different mechanisms of action. Substances such as marijuana and heroin mimic similar neurotransmitters, while amphetamines and cocaine stimulate the brain by prolonging the effect of dopamine. The duration of the drug's effect on the brain and the strength of its effect on the neural pathways play a very important role in the degree of addiction. Different ways of use, such as injecting or snorting, are also important components of effectiveness. That's why experts say heroin is the last drug you'll want to become addicted to because it is highly addictive.

Moreover, when drugs are not used, the person feels much more unhappy, depressed, nervous, and tense. Sometimes, depending on the withdrawal of the drug, they may feel sick and weak.

One of the biggest obstacles to addiction treatment is that dopamine is very closely related to memory. When dopamine is released, the environment that you are in is etched into memory and stays there for a long time. For example, if you see your friend, who you used to drink alcohol with, or a bar you went to years ago, you may suddenly have a craving for alcohol. As a result, even if you successfully complete addiction treatment, the environment you live in may remind you of your old life.

Data from neuroimaging studies also show that addiction causes significant changes in the brain. It is stated that people who use alcohol, cocaine, or morphine-derived drugs have a serious decrease in neurons in the prefrontal cortex (Kosten & George, 2002). This affects the decision-making mechanism and complicates the warning control.

It is a known fact that some people are more prone to addiction than others. Some people who smoke are addicted right away, some are not, and not everyone becomes addicted to morphine after surgery, just like not everyone who gambles is addicted. Experts state that many factors affect the addiction process, including genetics, the inadequacy of social support networks, trauma, and other mental problems.

However, one of the most important factors in addiction is age! According to a study conducted in 2014, it was observed that addicts who applied to treatment programs between the ages of 18-30 started substance use at the age of 17 and younger (Poudel & Gautam, 2017).

While there are studies that suggest DNA analysis can help determine the risk of addiction, most scientists agree that addiction is too complex of an issue to be solved by just analyzing genes. Education on mental health matters and addiction should be provided to children of all ages if we are looking to start solving our dopamine addiction problems as a society. It is of course easier to not burn your dopamine receptors than to try to fix it but there are ways to reconstruct the boost of your favorite neurotransmitter.

There are some ways to start rebuilding your dopamine receptors safely and naturally. Maintaining a safe level is up to you and is very important. You can try some of the methods below after your detox to slowly introduce healthy behaviors for dopamine production.

- Consume protein-rich foods

You can fill this deficiency by consuming plenty of protein-rich amino acids, specifically one that increases the level of dopamine, tyrosine. Examples of foods rich in tyrosine are beef, eggs, milk, legumes, and soy.

- Reduce consumption of foods containing saturated fat

Foods containing saturated fat, such as butter, whole milk, and coconut oil, have a property that disrupts dopamine signals in the brain. Therefore, you need to consume these foods as little as possible.

- Eat prebiotic foods

Bacteria living in the intestines directly contribute to the production of dopamine. Consuming foods like probiotic yogurt that support this production and are also good for mental health can help. There are a lot of flavors and types of prebiotics available in grocery stores these days. Kefir, yogurt, kombucha, and kimchi are all widely available in stores.

- Exercise regularly

It has been proven by scientific studies that aerobic exercises are effective in the treatment of Parkinson's disease (Oliveira de Carvalho et al., 2018). By taking at least 30 minute walks a day and exercising, you can avoid the diseases that are caused by a lack of dopamine.

- Get a generous amount of sunlight

Especially in the winter months, people who do not get enough sunlight may experience mood disorders. You may have heard the term "seasonal depression". Fresh air and the boost of vitamin D will definitely make you feel the effects of dopamine. However, you should avoid sun exposure between 10 am and 2 pm as the UV rays might be dangerous.

- Vitamins and minerals

You can increase the amount of dopamine you produce by taking magnesium, iron, folate, and/or vitamin B6 supplements. At the same time, you can eliminate a dopamine deficiency by consuming 2 cups of green tea a day. However, before you start using vitamin supplements, you should definitely have a blood test and consult a doctor, especially if you are a recovering addict or taking medication.

What causes an excess of dopamine?

In addition to the person's brain structure and genetic factors, neurobiology can also cause an excess of dopamine. Problems in the transmission of signals by neurotransmitters between nerves can lead to increased secretion of dopamine.

Does dopamine excess cause anxiety?

Dopamine dependency can cause many mental health problems and yes, it can cause anxiety. In this case, doctors usually prescribe anti-depressant drugs to slow down the excessive secretion of dopamine. However, these drugs are known to have side effects of extreme sluggishness and sleepiness.

Drugs containing dopamine are used in the treatment of which diseases?

Drugs containing dopamine can be prescribed for the treatment of many mental health diseases such as social phobia, depression, psychosis, DHEB, and especially Parkinson's disease.

Dopamine and serotonin

Both chemicals made by the brain are determinative of a person's mood and mental health. Known as the happiness hormone, serotonin, like dopamine, affects a person's mood, sleep pattern, menstrual cycle, and appetite. The low amount of serotonin may be behind depression and some mood disorders. However, serotonin does not have any role in the loss of movement control (Parkinson's).

Dopamine addiction or dopamine dependency?

Although dopamine often does not cause addiction on its own, excessive production of dopamine can lead to an addiction to the substance that helped produce the dopamine. The pleasure from alcohol and drug use redirects the brain in the direction of drug and alcohol use again. This situation can also vary depending on whether the person can control their desires and impulses. Depression, fatigue, and general dissatisfaction is commonly related to lower production of dopamine. Psychological depression can cause the person to turn to activities that make them feel happy and relaxed, such as alcohol, drugs, gambling, and sometimes even shopping.

Drugs for the Determined

In addiction treatment, change can be defined by the person's ability to control the desire for the substance they use, to continue a regular life, to cope with negative events without alcohol or substance, to have the power to cope with stress, and the ability to control negative emotions, in addition to stopping the use of the substance forever.

Addiction treatment is done in several parts, one of which includes a possible period of counteractive drugs to combat the addiction. While this should be done only by a doctor's recommendation and prescription, with the doctor following your treatment journey closely, it is still possible to fall back into your old habits if you are not being careful.

The usual procedure of addiction treatment is as follows. The first step is treatment during the withdrawal period. This can be as simple as a dopamine detox or as lengthy as a hospital stay, depending on the person's habits. This ensures that the effects of the substance pass and the physical or psychological problems that may be related to them are facilitated and overcome. Medical assistance is usually required during this cleansing period. Then, drug therapy, psychological support, and group treatments are applied for maintenance treatment and to prevent relapse. In this process, social support like the love and interest of family and the environment is very important.

The use of medication during the treatment of addiction is common but still controversial. Sometimes, these medications include addicting agents themselves and can cause severe long-term damage to the body. We will look into some drugs that are used in addiction treatment and talk about why you should have reasonable expectations and also should be wary of the side effects of each drug.

- Disulfiram

Disulfiram (Antabuse) is used to treat alcohol dependence. The main purpose is to create an unpleasant effect on the person taking disulfiram, even when only small amounts of alcohol are consumed. It treats alcohol dependence through negative reinforcement or aversion. Basically, disulfiram causes you to feel nearly immediate hangover symptoms after drinking alcohol. Vomiting, nausea, headaches, and breathlessness are all included.

By making you disgusted with alcohol, your body develops a serious reluctance against it. Disulfiram treatment should be combined with treatments such as psychotherapy, group therapy, and support groups such as Alcoholics Anonymous.

The severity of the disulfiram-alcohol reaction varies from patient to patient. In people with cardiovascular disease or those who are already highly intoxicated, disulfiram can cause major side effects like significant respiratory depression, cardiovascular collapse, myocardial infarction, convulsions, and death. Therefore, disulfiram is contraindicated in those with significant pulmonary or cardiovascular disease.

Disulfiram side-effects beyond an aversion to alcohol may include some fatigue, dermatitis, impotence, optic neuritis, various mental changes, and liver damage. However, these are rarely occurring.

The patient should be advised not to use any alcohol-containing substances, for example, cough drops, any kind of tonic, alcohol-based mouthwash, and alcohol-containing foods and sauces. Since some reactions have been observed in those who use alcohol-based aftershave or even inhale its vapor, clear reminders should be hung up around your living spaces to avoid any product containing alcohol, such as perfume.

- Naltrexone

This drug binds to and inhibits opiate receptors and helps relieve pain. These are the same receptors to which morphine, heroin, and other opiate substances bind. The main use of naltrexone is to consistently reverse opiate toxicity or to provide chronic treatment in opiate addiction.

Naltrexone is one of the drugs used in the treatment of alcoholics and drug addicts to keep them clean. It suppresses the body's opioid system, which regulates pain and plays a role in cell growth, repair, and inflammation.

- Buprenorphine and Methadone

Opioid addiction is one of the biggest health and social problems in the world, affecting all cultures, creating social problems, affecting the health status of the individual, and causing death. There are multiple options for the treatment of opiate addiction. Buprenorphine and Methadone are the two main and most effective agents used in the treatment of opioid addiction. Although both agents are structurally similar to each other, they have advantages as well as disadvantages in their use. When these drugs are used correctly, they reduce addicts' desire to use opiates. Methadone and Buprenorphine are seen as safer options for the treatment of addiction to opiates, as the likelihood of an overdose is low.

Both Methadone and Buprenorphine have been shown to be more effective than any other type of treatment for opioid addiction, especially when used in conjunction with psychosocial interventions.

- Prozac

Prozac is a type of antidepressant known as a selective serotonin reuptake inhibitor (SSRI). Prozac, the active ingredient of which is fluoxetine, is often used in the treatment of depression, and sometimes in the treatment of obsessive-compulsive disorder, premenstrual syndrome, and bulimia (eating disorder). It is a prescription drug and is available in many countries. It has fewer side effects than the old antidepressants. Nausea, headache, and trouble sleeping are common. However, these side effects are usually mild and pass within a few weeks. You cannot stop using Prozac once you start to feel better. In order not to experience side effects, you should stop taking the drug step-by-step under the supervision of a doctor.

Prozac is often prescribed to people during the treatment of addiction. Without dopamine, a person is not happy nor motivated to do anything. These can be seen as a sign of depression too as drug addiction recovery can cause someone to have depression and anxiety.

As with all antidepressant drugs, antidepressants containing the active ingredient fluoxetine are not drugs to be discontinued as soon as you feel well. It is important that the person finds a doctor they trust and follow their treatment plan profusely. The doctor will decide whether the person's disease is treated or not and will gradually reduce the dose until it is time to completely stop taking the medicine.

- Xanax

Xanax (alprazolam) is a psychiatric drug used as a sedative. It relieves severe attacks of fear and anxiety by acting on chemicals in the brain. It is used for a short time as it carries the risk of addiction. If gotten off suddenly without the doctor's knowledge, it can lead to withdrawal symptoms such as severe anxiety, confusion, and insomnia. For this reason, when the treatment ends, the drug is gradually discontinued, only under the control of the doctor. Xanax should never be taken with alcohol. In addition, simultaneous use with drugs can cause a narcotic effect, which can be literally fatal. The most common side effects are depression, drowsiness, forgetfulness, and balance and speech disorders. The drug should be taken in accordance with the doctor's instructions and should not be used for malicious purposes.

- Ambien

Zolpidem, also known as Ambien, is used to treat insomnia. It's effective within 3 hours after entering the body. It is a hypnotic drug that was originally approved by the FDA (American Food and Drug Administration) in 1992. It is one of the most prescribed hypnotics in the United States. It belongs to the group of sedative-hypnotic drugs and is used to reduce the function/activity of the brain. It helps individuals who have difficulty falling asleep and returning to sleep shortly after waking up. Like any drug, it must be eliminated from the body over time. The drug can take a toll on your kidneys in the long run.

- Klonopin

Klonopin is a prescription oral medication used to treat a variety of mental health disorders such as anxiety, panic disorder, and depression. However, because the drug has anticonvulsant properties, it is also prescribed to relieve seizures associated with epilepsy, as well as the symptoms of restless legs syndrome. Klonopin, a member of the benzodiazepine family of psychotropic drugs, is a mood-altering agent that targets the central nervous system. The biochemical action in the brain is what gives the drug the ability to influence perception and behavior. Unfortunately, this attribute is also what causes the deliberate misuse of this substance.

Like other psychotropic drugs, there are some risks associated with taking Klonopin. First, there may be a danger of developing a chemical addiction from prolonged or habitual use. This risk appears to be particularly pronounced when this drug is used repeatedly to counteract insomnia. However, when used responsibly and under the guidance of a professional healthcare practitioner, the potential benefits can outweigh this risk.

At the other end of the spectrum is the issue of pullbacks. It is absolutely important to "wean" the patient from this drug in ascending stages. Otherwise, severe anxiety and irritability may occur. In fact, stopping this medication suddenly and completely can cause psychotic episodes, including dysphoria (depression) and hallucinations. Additionally, sporadic seizures may occur even in those who have experienced nothing before taking the drug.

- Adderall

Adderall is an amphetamine prescribed by doctors for the treatment of Attention deficit hyperactivity disorder and narcolepsy. This drug can also be used in some cases of severe depression. It was first launched in the 1920s under the name Obetrol. It is a prescription drug and should be because it is easy to abuse and often is.

Adderall was introduced as a water-soluble tablet in 1997 and contains various amphetamine salts. Its main active ingredient is dextroamphetamine and racemic amphetamine salts.

This drug, which is released for people with a lack of attention and focus, is of course also used for bad purposes. There are also people who put themselves in a very dangerous position by consuming Adderall with alcohol.

It is also possible that this drug, for which a documentary called *Take Your Pills* was made, causes a serious addiction when used unnecessarily and continuously. It is said that addiction to the drug makes even ordinary activities impossible without the use of the drug after a while. It was stated that this drug, which was prescribed to 16 million people in 2012 alone, required rehabilitation due to addiction in 116,000 people (*Take Your Pills* | Netflix Official Site, 2019).

In summary, although it is a very useful drug for those who need it, it is very, very easy to abuse. Therefore, if you have trouble focusing, it would be best to seek medical support outside of Adderall.

Chapter 3: Balancing Comfort and Discomfort

Sometimes, we do things just to comfort ourselves even if it is not necessary. Have you ever checked what a word means in the dictionary even though you already know? Or have you ever set a timer for something only to end up checking the time every 30 seconds in case you miss it? These are all anxious behaviors we all have that provide an extra layer of comfort for us. However, this layer of comfort can sometimes keep us in a prison called "the comfort zone".

The truth is, in order to become the best version of yourself, you must push through your own limits. This often means staying away from comfort and actually letting yourself experience discomfort.

Comfort and discomfort are closely related despite meaning the opposite of each other. You can find comfort in your discomfort and vice versa. There is a difference between not wanting to be comfortable and not being comfortable out of your own control. Oftentimes, self-healing techniques are overlooked when it comes to anxiety and depression.

What is Anxiety?

Anxiety has become one of the number one mental health problems in the world. Generalized anxiety disorder affects millions of people worldwide, and that number continues to rise at an alarming rate. But the good news is that there are many techniques you can use to effectively manage anxiety. Anxiety after suffering an addiction can be severe and be accompanied by its best friend, depression. Not knowing how to spend your day after recovery, being anxious about all the bridges you've burned during addiction, and the financial worry of your future can all pile up to be very anxiety-inducing.

People organize their lives by making plans for the future. Worrying about the future is a way for the human mind to protect itself. However, the exacerbation of this situation increases the rate of stress and anxiety, causing you to feel constantly under threat. It is important to seek help from a professional when you start to feel worse. But at this point, there are a few things you can do in your daily life as well.

Trying to combat anxiety

Anxiety feeds on itself. If you let negative thoughts grow, you may end up feeling crazy. Anxiety can pile up like a snowball rolling down a hill and you are the only one with the power to stop it. First, you must learn to stop negative thoughts. This means identifying thoughts as they arise. When you find yourself feeding your intrusive thoughts, ask yourself, "Is this really likely to happen?" Stop thinking about the past and the future and try to imagine what your life would be like if you didn't have worries.

If that doesn't work, make a list. Write down what's on your mind and what you've done about it. This writing exercise will help you rationalize problems and find their true size. In other words, it won't let them continue to grow and spin around in your head.

You can also write down your goals and how you will achieve them.

Happiness and discomfort

The brain messenger dopamine regulates feelings of happiness. Researchers now know that it also has a great influence on fear. The neurotransmitter dopamine plays a key role in the development of fear in the brain. Researchers at the Technical University of Aachen have shown that anxious people have particularly high concentrations of dopamine in the amygdala region of the brain (Klasen et al., 2019). This knowledge could help develop new therapeutic approaches for anxiety disorders. Let's look into it a little deeper.

Dopamine has traditionally been attributed to feelings such as joyful expectations. It is also known that a reduced amount of dopamine in the brainstem is the cause of movement disorders in Parkinson's patients. In brain examinations, researchers have now shown that anxious people have higher dopamine concentrations in the amygdala when looking at frightening, anxiety-inducing images (Oscar Berman et al., 2008). They also discovered that an intensive exchange of the amygdala and anterior cingulum reduced anxiety.

"The more the areas of the brain communicated with each other, the lower the activity of the amygdala when it came to perceiving anxiety-inducing stimuli," says psychiatrist Gerhard Gründer (Wolff et al., 2020). According to the doctor, this can be used therapeutically: "In psychotherapy, patients can learn to control their fear perception over the long term by changing their behavior" (Wolff et al., 2020).

Dopamine for fear

Classic behavioral trauma therapy exposes patients to repeated stimuli that are reminiscent of the trauma. The aim is to unlearn the connection between the two and thus get rid of the fear. A well-known drug can help the brain on jumps, as researchers from the German Resilience Center at the University of Mainz discovered.

Exposure therapy is based on erasing the link between stimulus and fear response. But to do this, the new learning experiences would have to be permanently memorized, explains the first author of the publication Anna Gerlicher (Lonsdorf et al., 2019). It is already known that spontaneous activity in the frontal lobe contributes to this and that this in turn depends on the neuronal messenger substance dopamine. The idea of Gerlicher and her colleagues was to raise the dopamine level with a drug to support the learning process.

To do this, the team initially taught 40 men to be afraid of a geometric symbol. If it appeared on the screen, they received a painful electric shock every second time on average - but not if another symbol appeared. The researchers tested the fear response they had learned by measuring the test subjects' skin conductivity, among other things. On the following day, the test subjects were presented with both symbols again, but without shock treatment. You should now find that both symbols are harmless, similar to exposure to therapeutic therapy. Using functional magnetic resonance imaging, the researchers tracked the activity in the subjects' brains 10, 45, and 90 minutes after exposure (Whitten, 2012).

Half of the test persons swallowed 150 milligrams of the dopamine precursor levodopa immediately after the harmless experience with the fearful symbol

(L-Dopa) is also used in Parkinson's disease. Compared to participants who had received a dummy drug, the fear response to the critical symbol was weaker in the test subjects who had been given L-dopa. In addition, three-quarters of an hour after the confrontation, certain patterns of neuronal activity spontaneously appeared in the ventromedial prefrontal cortex - and the more so, the less anxious the participants had reacted to the symbol.

According to the researchers, the frontal lobe becomes active whenever an expectation is not fulfilled, such as painful shock in the case of the learned fear response. If the dopamine level is increased, the new learning experience can be better remembered. What has not been researched, however, is when exactly the intake of L-Dopa should take place in order to achieve an optimal effect (Morse, 2006).

Dealing with discomfort

How can you change something in your life when you are absolutely terrified of it? And how can you get into action and actually do it despite your fear? Unfortunately, there is no one-size-fits-all solution for this and you must simply keep trying to find a way that suits you!

But a simple strategy can make things a lot easier for you.

The Home Called Comfort Zone

We all have our so-called comfort zones. In other words, the area in which we feel safe and comfortable. Oftentimes, we are reluctant to leave this area.

Sometimes, however, you come into situations in life that present you with a challenge. You ask yourself, "Do I dare to change? Do I keep feeling sorry for myself for my past mistakes and bad decisions, or do I rise from the ashes and become a whole new person?" Hopefully, your answer to these is to actually do something about the way you feel.

The comfort zone is really difficult to leave. The secure job, the well-established partnership, the house that has already been half financed, or the bad habits you can't seem to do without, all need a very solid reason to change. The number one solid reason behind any of these can be growth! We grow beyond our wildest imaginations when we step out of our comfort zone.

To be afraid of it is more than understandable. Because none of us like to lose anything. And "out of the comfort zone" means "risk". A risk of not feeling the same, comfortable way you have been feeling, a risk of having to work hard to better your life when your life right now doesn't seem so bad. So it is only logical that you will find it difficult to leave your comfort zone.

Personal development, spiritual growth, and life lessons are often found right outside of your comfort zone, which we call the safe zone. You struggle with the challenges of the outside world and dare to make mistakes. Even if your mind is trying to keep you in your safe space to protect you, it's still up to you to get out.

Safety, familiarity, convenience. These are just a few terms that describe how you might feel when you're within the confines of your safe space. As long as you avoid uncertainty and fixate on habits you already know, you won't have to be judged, you won't have to worry about the new, will you? This is understandable as people tend to live by their routines. Understandable but deep down you know that personality development, spiritual growth, and life lessons are often found outside of your safe space. Outside of this area, you take the risk of struggling and failing. You are a little hesitant and timid, but you try your luck. Because the beauty of life's gifts often come in the most uncomfortable situations.

Okay, some people prefer to step out and do different things more than others. Because each of us has a different attitude towards risk. Some people like to play and look for risks. Others prefer to play it safe. You too have your own "default". People who suffer from addiction often choose to not do much about it because doing something about it would mean giving up the drugs, therefore, no dopamine. Even though it is hard, one must push themselves to find the boundaries of their comfort zone before stepping completely outside of it. This step-by-step approach will make it easier to give it a go.

Comfort zone = golden cage?

The comfort zone also offers you a lot of security and habits you have come to love. Why should you give up all of this for the uncertainty? Here is why, when you swap comfortable life for "no idea what's coming", you learn and experience new things.

If you think that would be stupid, just think to yourself, do you always want to carry on like now? Can you really imagine that? Is that going to let you live your best life? Are you truly your happiest self? It is okay if you don't have solid answers to these. The questions can get really deep.

Actually, a question that many of us don't want to ask ourselves would be, what if you don't want to go on like this? The honest answer to that could be frightening.

If you come to this conclusion, "I actually know that I cannot and will not go on like this," then you may notice right away how your heart drops at the thought. Because you may not dare to really do it, because you're scared of making a big mistake, because you basically avoid risk like the devil avoids holy water, because the insecurity won't let you sleep at night, or because you would like change most of all, but without risk or pain.

Once you get to the point where you think, "Actually, I don't want to do it anymore ...," from this moment the ring is open. The ring for the struggle between your desire for security and your desire for change. And if you don't want to continue as before, then that means this: You will have to leave your comfort zone soon one way or another. But how are you supposed to do that?

Fear leads to self-sabotage

When you are afraid of leaving your comfort zone, it often leads to behavior patterns that will not get you anywhere:

- The Fearful Refusal: deep down you want to change. But you are so afraid of your own courage that you prefer to suppress your wishes by all means and remain unhappy.
- The Skillful Ignorance: You know you want the change. But you are afraid of the consequences. So don't think

about it any further. Better to forget. And keep running away.
- The Infinite Yes but not Now: You see the need for change, but think to yourself, "I am not going to run from this but I can do it some other time instead of now." This thought continues until the person either takes action or dies.
- The Eternal Wailing: You are dissatisfied, but you don't lift a finger yourself. You prefer to wait until something magical happens and things get fixed on their own. It is almost like everyone and everything else is responsible for your lack of happiness but yourself.
- The Airy Dreaming: You make big plans and like to talk about them a lot. But after you finish talking, little or nothing happens. Dreaming is your refuge, but you do not act.
- The Perfect Preparation: You roll over books and attend seminars and forge plans after plans. So you have the feeling that you are doing something, but you always stay in your safe area.
- The Wild Jumping Around: Some days you want this but some days something completely different. Every day you run in your new favorite direction. This is how you always start but never go any further. And in the end, you go around in circles.

These are all behavior patterns that ensure that you can lull yourself to safety. These patterns keep you in your comfort zone or maybe the term "trap" would be a better one in this scenario.

Are you in the comfort zone out of fear of loss?

Maybe you recognize yourself in one of these behaviors. But that's not that bad. These are behaviors that are supposed to protect you. So they're actually something good. They only stand in your way when you really want change. Staying in your comfort zone has its place. You can stay there. Nobody can force you to go out, fight for your happiness, and get a bloody nose in the process. The decisive factor at this point is your demands on yourself. Whether you say, "I would rather have the same exact life regardless of how taxing it is." That is perfectly fine. It's entirely in the vein of, "He who is poor in desires is rich". Or you could instead say, "I want more out of my life, and for that I also accept stumbling, bruises, and pain." If you tend towards the latter, then the question inevitably arises:

"How do I get out of my comfort zone?"

- Design the change process yourself

If you want to change, it is important that you take it into your own hands and shape it in such a way that you can endure it. It's similar to doing sports. If you want to be able to lift 200 pounds, but you can only do 100 pounds today, you wouldn't start off your challenge by trying to lift 200 pounds. You wouldn't be able to do it, wouldn't have fun, and could even hurt yourself in the process. Overloading yourself doesn't make sense. And you can apply this principle to very many areas of life, including even in your comfort zone.

In concrete terms, this means that you don't have to leave your current situation or go from 0 to 100 immediately, but you can do it slowly and with mini-steps that won't hurt you. That way you can proceed according to the level of difficulty and not have to start with the hardest part right away.

Yes, that sounds pretty logical and simple at first. But how many people really do it that way? Or to put it the other way round: If you really would do it like this, what are you still afraid of? Maybe it's not what you are doing to change but the size of the change itself.

But that's the charm of this approach. You stay in a "safe zone" for a very long time, where you can turn around at any time.

- Have a clear strategy out of the comfort zone

Imagine that you are dissatisfied with your job. So dissatisfied that you realize: Yes, I want to change. It makes me unhappy. But you don't really want to quit either. After all, you have a house to pay off and children to feed. Uh-oh. How would you get out of this situation? No one likes to have crisis conversations with their boss. Not the simplest of solutions, which in turn leads to you putting it off, ignoring it, complaining about it, or sinking into daydreams (see the list above). Instead, what could a mini-step that doesn't hurt you look like? This is how you get into action: A mini step means going from 0 to 1 on the scale. That is the goal. So if you are dissatisfied with your job, you could, for example, take a pen and piece of paper and write down what your complaints are. Write down the things that make you unhappy about your current situation. It's a step that doesn't cost you anything, just a little time and paper. But it's a small first step. In which you record for yourself what exactly is going on.

What could be another such mini-step?

Next, you need to slowly map out what you want to do and how you want to do it. There are tons of mini-steps like this that you can take one at a time without ever having to step out of your comfort zone.

When it comes to decisions that are harder like leaving addiction behind, the same analogy still applies but the steps might need to be bigger depending on the addiction and the person's health.

Here is a simple guide to how to take the mini-steps:

- Analyze your problem
- Think about where you would actually prefer to go with your plan
- Clarify your "why" so that you gain clarity for yourself and can read it over if you ever lose sight of your goal
- Make all possible options clear and continue to have a conversation with yourself about the possibility of changing options
- Set your own deadlines/commit yourself to something
- To make a decision last, you must become completely captivated by the idea of realizing your goal
- Think about your first mini-goal and go with the one that scares you the least

Meditation for anxiety relief

By now, most know that meditation has been used for centuries to calm the mind, better manage stress and anxiety, and find inner peace. While it's great to know that the older generations found it useful and passed it along, there was no way of proving the benefits of meditation to the skeptics in the West. Without science, it could have very well been brushed off as an old wives tale.

Thanks to great scientists who were intrigued by the practice, we have more and more scientific studies proving that meditation is not just a great way to heal mental issues but also a great way to decrease the symptoms of some physical illnesses like high blood pressure, poor digestion, and sleep issues. Often, physical illnesses are created or worsened by mental issues like anxiety, stress, and depression.

Best meditation types for anxiety

When anxiety takes over, our minds can't seem to focus on anything else other than the fact that there is something wrong. Sometimes we don't even know what is causing the anxiety and that ends up making it worse. With these meditation techniques, you can redirect your focus from the anxious feelings to a calmer, clearer state of mind.

Traka Meditation: Traka Meditation helps you focus on one thing at a time, helping you relax. The first thing is to choose an object around the room you are in to focus your eyes on. Throughout your entire session, your eyes and mind should be on this object, only thinking about things about the item. Your eyes and mind will be focused on your item and every thought and worry that distracts you will eventually fade away. Every time you find yourself distracted, simply bring your attention back to the item you had picked. While meditating, your brain will enjoy the quiet and reward it with releasing the GABA chemical, which is known as the 'calm neurotransmitter'. This chemical will slow down your racing heart rate, and even help you get to sleep better if you are in the mood for a nap.

Mantra Meditation: Choosing a mantra that works for you and completely focusing on it forces your body into a total state of relaxation. The number one enemy of anxiety is racing thoughts and a constant state of worry. Mantras like "Aum" that have a positive meaning will help you become more aware of the positive possibilities that are yet to come than the negativity that's currently holding you hostage.

Best meditation types for depression

Meditation is one of the best ways to prevent depression, as well as reduce the symptoms of it for those who have it. Depression has a stronger chemical effect on the brain than a lot of people realize. A depressed brain doesn't release enough of the necessary chemicals for us to be able to experience pleasure, relaxation, or happiness. Studies have found that meditation helps release those important chemicals in depressed brains and help the healing process. More active meditation types might be better for people with depression to prevent the mind from sinking into negative thoughts during the session. The following types of meditation have been clinically proven to help depressed people.

Loving- Kindness Meditation: Depression sometimes causes a person to be harsher on themselves and others. Positive feelings and thoughts seem so infrequent that focusing on the negative seems to be the only way. LKM helps the meditator have fewer negative thoughts while increasing their mood. This meditation technique has been proven to train the brain to have more compassion towards yourself and others, reduce self-ridicule, and increase the amount of serotonin in the brain.

Yoga Meditation: Yoga is a form of mental and physical exercise. The poses are physically demanding while breathing and focusing on your balance is taking your mind away from anything disruptive. The reason why physical exercise is recommended to people with depression is that when you do something physically demanding, your brain rewards itself with good chemicals like endorphins, which are known as pain-killer chemicals; dopamine, known as the feel-good chemical; and serotonin, the happy-chemical. Studies show that self-awareness yoga, also known as Kundalini yoga, in particular, helps manage fear, anger, and negative thoughts.

Tantra Meditation: It might be difficult for depressed people to say something positive about themselves. Tantra teaches self-love and awareness. By the end of the meditation session, the brain can physically feel the positivity and light the meditation has generated. The nerve cells in the body will be bathing in serotonin and dopamine, creating a happier mood that will last.

Keeping a meditation journal

Therapists keep notes on their patients and their progress by making notes on a piece of paper during each session. They compare each new session to the older one to see if there is any progress, if some issues have gotten worse, or if they need to readjust their technique. By keeping a meditation journal after each time you are done meditating, you can keep an eye on your progress and see the results of meditating easier. When you first start your meditation journey, it will take a while to see the results and you might end up missing the small things like your thought patterns changing or being less distracted. A meditation journal doesn't take much time and can be a wonderful tool to keep an eye on your progress.

- The Benefits

The point of a journal is not to see if you are getting the results you wanted or not but rather to see the changes you had over time, motivating you to keep meditating. It will help you develop a better-tailored practice for you by giving you some hindsight into your meditation journey. When you decide to start meditating, you might have some ideas on what you want out of it but your meditation map will basically be blank. Keeping a journal can show you where you were and where you are headed so you can make the necessary adjustments with things like the duration, style, or technique of your practice. Seeing how far you've come since starting can also inspire you to become more social and take up new hobbies.

- How to Start?

Get an empty notebook and keep it right with your meditation cushion. You can leave the journal on your cushion when you are done to always have it near and put it next to your cushion when you are meditating. When you sit on your cushion and consider what thoughts and emotions you have brought to your practice that day, make a mental note of them and keep on with your practice. After you are done, pick up your journal and make your entry. Repeat after each session.

- What to Write?

If you can't seem to write as much today as you did after yesterday's session, it does not mean you didn't meditate properly today. You don't need a specific structure to keep a journal and forcing yourself to stick to a word count or structure can lead to feelings of failure. It doesn't need to take a lot of time nor does it need to look pretty. As long as you can understand it, it can be as casual as you want.

Write down the day, time, the type of meditation you practiced, and the duration of your session, and then write freely about how you felt before, during, and after your practice. Meditation doesn't feel the same every single day so it is also okay to make brief notes about your practice one day and write a 2 paragraph essay another day. You can use some of these examples until you figure out which works the best for you.

Why Spirituality is Important

Spirituality talks about ego and selfishness. It suggests that there is no selfless good deed in life. You might think "I gave that homeless person $20. How is me being $20 poorer so he can eat, selfish?" and the answer is that while it is not selfish, it also isn't selfless. Helping that homeless person made you feel good, did it not? You get a boost of dopamine when you engage in spiritual activities that feed your soul on a much deeper level than anything else.

Every good deed we do comes back to us as a positive feeling. This may sound crooked but it is okay to feel good about yourself as long as you help others and realize that we are all one. Even science supports this theory. Meditation styles like Loving-Kindness Meditation have been proven to increase our compassion towards other people and make us happier people during the process. One of the things spirituality focuses on is letting go of your ego and realizing how small you are in the universe while still being a part of everything that connects it together. Practicing spirituality and meditation can help you understand your surroundings, the people around you, and the world better, leading to a more sustainably happy and anxiety-free life.

The Depression-Discomfort Defense

Experienced anxieties cause hopelessness, and constant anxiety causes tremendous fatigue. As a result of hopelessness and fatigue, reluctance and finally depression appear. So roughly speaking, our brains become depressed to avoid severe anxiety. It transitions from over-struggling to pacification. Serious uncertainty about the future (anxiety) lends itself to absolute negativity (depression). Because the human mind cannot bear uncertainty, it seeks clarity.

The causes of depression are very diverse and there is no single cause. In some cases, it may occur due to an existing physical disease or medication used by the person. This condition is called secondary depression. Depression is not a simple disease; it is a disease in which medical evaluation is extremely important and requires diagnosis and treatment by psychiatrists.

Dangers of avoiding

One of the reasons for wanting to withdraw into one's own shell rather than enter unknown territory is the fear of the unknown. Avoiding situations in which you are unsure can relieve your stress or anxiety in the short term. But research from 2011 published in the Journal of Counseling and Clinical Psychology shows that prolonged avoidance behavior can actually trigger much higher levels of stress (Newman & Llera, 2011). The researchers tested 1211 participants in their late middle age 3 times over 10 years and investigated the relationship between stressful avoidance, acute and chronic stress triggers, and depression symptoms. After four years, they found a significant relationship between avoidance behavior and stress triggers. Moreover, after 10 years, they were discovered to be linked to symptoms of depression (McLean et al., 2015).

Perception or reality

According to a study conducted by researchers from the University of London Academy in 2016, you may find situations where you do not know the outcome and this is more stressful than situations where you know will have a bad outcome (Bhui et al., 2016). In the study, it was stated that a group of participants would be given an electric shock with a 50% probability, a group would definitely be exposed to electricity, and a group would definitely not be exposed to it. Participants with a 50% probability were exposed to higher stress than those who would definitely receive a shock (not surprisingly, those who would not receive a shock were also less stressed). On the bright side, those with the highest stress response to the unknown were the best predictors of whether they would be shocked. This showed that stress can increase risk assessment ability. Researchers have provided numerous real-life examples to which these findings can be applied. For example, in a job interview, you will be most comfortable if you are sure that you will or will not be hired, while you will be more anxious if you are in doubt. The concern here lies in the uncertainty itself. In other words, in the fear of the unknown.

Horror

An article published in the Journal of Anxiety Disorders in 2016 examined the criteria that trigger our most basic fears (National Institute of Mental Health, 2019). Researchers have suggested that the fear of the unknown may be the most fundamental fear behind all other fears. This uncertainty not only creates anxiety and affects psychological disorders, but is also effective in our daily emotions and decision mechanisms.

After reading the above research, you may wish to dampen this fear completely. "I will step into real life and stop feeling this fear," you might think. This idea will fail for two reasons:

1) You cannot get rid of fear through thinking. You may think you are brave with all your might, but the only real way to be free from fears is to be exposed to them. In other words, the way to deal with them is to experience them.

2) You need fear to survive. Although you often feel that it is working against you, it is actually on your side and constantly works to protect you. Without fear, you may find yourself in the midst of situations that endanger your health and safety. Your stress response serves to protect you.

Obscurity

You may think that the obstacle to facing real life is your stress response. According to a 2018 study that looked at people's basic responses to uncertainty, the real hurdle is how you perceive that stress (UCL, 2018). Researchers have found that the stress of the unknown is always present, yet the stress decreases when you perceive your situation as safe. When you're worried about your safety, even without danger, your stress response is activated, which can contribute to chronic stress and other health problems. The feeling of being safe in different situations can be gained by being exposed to these situations.

If you live the same every day, your brain, which carries the archive of your past and is shaped by your past, means that you're trapped in a routine. That means you are actually living in the past. Everything is the same, everything is predictable, and everything is old. No change means being doomed to live the life of the person you are dissatisfied with. The dungeon of the soul burning with the passion of liberation...

To dream is to build the future. The changing mind gets rid of the past with the dream of new ideas and focuses on the future. Positive thoughts, that is, being hopeful about the future, lead us to live in the present. Because if there were negative thoughts, we would call it future anxiety. But positive thinking does not allow us to lie down and stare at the sky to dream of our wonderful future but to go with the flow to build that future.

Unfortunately, the events we were exposed to in our infancy when we were all creatures that could not think yet, created our emotional world. These emotions, which are the lowest bricks of the unconscious, are like the building blocks of the thoughts and behaviors of the human consciousness. So this is the first spark of the cycle; Belief born out of feelings has given shape to the mind that gives birth to thoughts. However, the adult individual, as a conscious being, observes that their mind, a significant part of which has already been formed, changes beliefs.

Negative thoughts send messages to our bodies, changing our chemistry. The body gets stressed by the negative messages of thoughts and initiates physiological changes. The stress of our body triggers our thoughts to become even more negative. They have become a chain of reactions that we must break. As I explained above, no matter how negative or dire the current situation is; If we can think of a positive scenario for the future if we can believe that all this will pass, all the troubles we are experiencing will be alleviated. It becomes a burden we can lift. This prevents us from giving up.

Faith comes before thought. That belief will give us the strength to cope with difficulties is a fundamental construct and is part of our self-awareness. If we have this belief, our thoughts run our minds for a positive exit idea. Almost everything in life has a solution; sometimes it just isn't what we originally imagined. Our mind focused on positive thinking starts to produce solutions that will feed our belief this time.

When our thoughts change, our emotions come alive. Exciting emotions create new neurological connections (synapses) and generate bright ideas, positive thoughts, and exciting plans. We want and we take action to get what we want.

References

2-Minute Neuroscience: Dopamine. (2018). [YouTube Video]. In *YouTube.*

https://www.youtube.com/watch?v=Wa8_nLwQIpg

6 Strategies to Overcome Fear and Anxiety. (2018, June 21). Real Life Counseling. https://reallifecounseling.us/overcome-fear-and-anxiety/

Ambien: Is dependence a concern? (n.d.). Mayo Clinic. https://www.mayoclinic.org/diseases-conditions/insomnia/expert-answers/ambien/faq-20058103

Anxiety Treatment Methods - Womans Mirror. (n.d.). Womensmiror.com. Retrieved October 6, 2021, from https://womensmiror.com/anxiety-treatment-methods/

APA PsycNet. (n.d.). Psycnet.apa.org. Retrieved October 6, 2021, from https://psycnet.apa.org/record/2004-00216-001

Ashkenazy, S., & DeKeyser Ganz, F. (2019). The Differentiation Between Pain and Discomfort: A Concept Analysis of

Discomfort. *Pain Management Nursing.* https://doi.org/10.1016/j.pmn.2019.05.003

Ayano, G. (2016). Dopamine: Receptors, Functions, Synthesis, Pathways, Locations and Mental Disorders: Review of Literatures. *Journal of Mental Disorders and Treatment, 2*(2). https://doi.org/10.4172/2471-271x.1000120

Collier, R. (2018). A short history of pain management. *Canadian Medical Association Journal, 190*(1), E26–E27. https://doi.org/10.1503/cmaj.109-5523

Connolly, M. (2018, January 24). *Know the Difference Between Pain and Discomfort to Achieve Excellence.* Neways Somatic Psychotherapy & Coaching. https://newayscenter.com/2018/01/24/difference-between-pain-and-discomfort-achieve-excellence/

Cristol, H. (2019, June 19). *What Is Dopamine?* WebMD; WebMD. https://www.webmd.com/mental-health/what-is-dopamine

Detailed Anxiety, Stress and Related Illnesses, Disorders. (n.d.). Udemy. Retrieved October 6, 2021, from https://www.udemy.com/course/detailed-anxiety-stress-and-related-illnesses-disorders/

Disulfiram: MedlinePlus Drug Information. (2019, December). Medlineplus.gov.

https://medlineplus.gov/druginfo/meds/a682602.html

Dopamine deficiency: Symptoms, causes, and treatment. (2018, January 17). Www.medicalnewstoday.com.

https://www.medicalnewstoday.com/articles/320637#outlook

Drugs & Medications. (2019). Webmd.com. https://www.webmd.com/drugs/2/drug-7399/naltrexone-oral/details

Effects of Dopamine: How Dopamine Drives Human Behavior. (2019, September 5). Into Action Recovery Centers. https://www.intoactionrecovery.com/how-dopamine-drives-our-behavior/

Five effective ways to stop anxiety attacks. (2016, June 19). Bright Side — Inspiration. Creativity. Wonder. https://brightside.me/inspiration-psychology/five-effective-ways-to-stop-anxiety-attacks-181255/

Flow States and Creativity. (2014). Psychology Today. https://www.psychologytoday.com/us/blog/the-playing-field/201402/flow-states-and-creativity

good junk food snacks. (n.d.). Tikstation.com. Retrieved October 6, 2021, from https://tikstation.com/jcjk/good-junk-food-snacks

Information, A. (2021, February 20). *What Is Dopamine, Where Is It Produced, What Does It Do?* Allover Information. https://www.alloverinformation.com/what-is-dopamine-where-is-it-produced-what-does-it-do/

Juergens, J. (2013). *Adderall Addiction and Abuse - Prescription Amphetamines.* AddictionCenter. https://www.addictioncenter.com/stimulants/adderall/

Klonopin Addiction and Abuse - Clonazepam Abuse - Addiction Center. (n.d.). AddictionCenter. https://www.addictioncenter.com/benzodiazepines/klonopin/

Kotler, S. (2014, February 23). *Social Flow.* Medium. https://medium.com/@kotlersteven/social-flow-b04436fac167

Mission. (2017, November 29). *Why It's So Important to Seek Discomfort*. Mission.org. https://medium.com/the-mission/why-its-so-important-to-seek-discomfort-34fb2519a884#:~:text=Generally%20speaking%2C%20the%20benefits%20from

Opioids may slow down wound healing. (2017, March 5). McKnight's Long Term Care News. https://www.mcknights.com/news/opioids-may-slow-down-wound-healing#:~:text=Results%20showed%20that%20patients%20who

Pain Vs. Discomfort: How to know the difference and how to know when it's time to back off. (n.d.). Wild Heart Medicine. Retrieved October 6, 2021, from https://wildheartmedicine.com/blog/2020/4/27/pain-vs-discomfort-how-to-know-the-difference-and-how-to-know-when-its-time-to-back-off

Patel, S. (n.d.). *Why Feeling Uncomfortable Is The Key To Success*. Forbes. Retrieved October 6, 2021, from https://www.forbes.com/sites/sujanpatel/2016/03/09/wh

y-feeling-uncomfortable-is-the-key-to-success/?sh=45cf1d541913

PechaKucha 20x20. (n.d.). Www.pechakucha.com. Retrieved October 6, 2021, from https://www.pechakucha.com/presentations/psychologic-disorders

Pietrangelo, A. (2019, November 5). *Dopamine Effects on the Body, Plus Drug and Hormone Interactions*. Healthline. https://www.healthline.com/health/dopamine-effects

Prozac | Abuse, Side Effects, Detox, Withdrawal and Treatment. (n.d.). Nova Recovery Center near Austin Texas. https://novarecoverycenter.com/drugs/prozac/

Prozac Addiction. (n.d.). The Recovery Village Drug and Alcohol Rehab. https://www.therecoveryvillage.com/prozac-addiction/

Quick Tip--The Difference Between Pain and Discomfort. (2015, August 21). DizRuns.com. http://www.dizruns.com/difference-between-pain-and-discomfort/

SAMHSA. (2014, May 14). *National Helpline | SAMHSA - Substance Abuse and Mental Health Services Administration.* Samhsa.gov. https://www.samhsa.gov/find-help/national-helpline

Sugar Is a Drug and Here's How We're Hooked. (2013, September 18). Healthline. https://www.healthline.com/health-news/addiction-sugar-acts-like-drug-in-the-brain-and-could-lead-to-addiction-091813

What happens if you drink alcohol while taking naltrexone? (n.d.). Drugs.com. Retrieved October 6, 2021, from https://www.drugs.com/medical-answers/you-drink-alcohol-taking-naltrexone-3548694/

What Role Does Dopamine Play in Addiction? (2018, February 21). Inspire Malibu. https://www.inspiremalibu.com/blog/drug-addiction/dopamine-and-addiction/

Why Discomfort is Good and a Sign of Growth -. (2016, November 22). https://www.skilledatlife.com/why-discomfort-is-good-and-a-sign-of-growth/

Why Riding the Wave of Discomfort Is Good for You | Psychology Today. (n.d.). Www.psychologytoday.com. Retrieved October 6, 2021, from https://www.psychologytoday.com/us/blog/the-romance-work/201412/why-riding-the-wave-discomfort-is-good-you

wikiHow. (2018, March 31). *Increase Dopamine Sensitivity*. WikiHow; wikiHow. https://www.wikihow.com/Increase-Dopamine-Sensitivity

American Psychological Association. (2017, July). What Is Exposure Therapy? *Https://Www.apa.org*. https://www.apa.org/ptsd-guideline/patients-and-families/exposure-therapy

Bernard, S. A., Chelminski, P. R., Ives, T. J., & Ranapurwala, S. I. (2018). Management of Pain in the United States—A Brief History and Implications for the Opioid Epidemic. *Health Services Insights, 11*, 117863291881944. https://doi.org/10.1177/1178632918819440

Bhui, K., Dinos, S., Galant-Miecznikowska, M., de Jongh, B., & Stansfeld, S. (2016). Perceptions of work stress causes and effective interventions in employees working in public, private and non-governmental organisations: A qualitative study. *BJPsych Bulletin, 40*(6), 318–325. https://doi.org/10.1192/pb.bp.115.050823

Collier, R. (2018). A short history of pain management. *Canadian Medical Association Journal, 190*(1), E26–E27. https://doi.org/10.1503/cmaj.109-5523

Goldberg, D. S. (2017). Pain, objectivity and history: understanding pain stigma. *Medical Humanities, 43*(4), 238–243. https://doi.org/10.1136/medhum-2016-011133

Holahan, C. J., Moos, R. H., Holahan, C. K., Brennan, P. L., & Schutte, K. K. (2005). Stress Generation, Avoidance Coping, and Depressive Symptoms: A 10-Year Model. *Journal of Consulting and Clinical Psychology, 73*(4), 658–666. https://doi.org/10.1037/0022-006x.73.4.658

Klasen, M., Wolf, D., Eisner, P. D., Eggermann, T., Zerres, K., Zepf, F. D., Weber, R., & Mathiak, K. (2019). Serotonergic Contributions to Human Brain Aggression Networks. *Frontiers in Neuroscience, 13*. https://doi.org/10.3389/fnins.2019.00042

Kosten, T. R., & George, T. P. (2002). The neurobiology of opioid dependence: implications for treatment. *Science & Practice Perspectives*, *1*(1), 13–20. https://www.ncbi.nlm.nih.gov/pmc/articles/PMC2851054/

Lonsdorf, T. B., Klingelhöfer-Jens, M., Andreatta, M., Beckers, T., Chalkia, A., Gerlicher, A., Jentsch, V. L., Meir Drexler, S., Mertens, G., Richter, J., Sjouwerman, R., Wendt, J., & Merz, C. J. (2019). Navigating the garden of forking paths for data exclusions in fear conditioning research. *ELife*, *8*, e52465. https://doi.org/10.7554/eLife.52465

McLean, C. P., Su, Y.-J., Carpenter, J. K., & Foa, E. B. (2015). Changes in PTSD and Depression During Prolonged Exposure and Client-Centered Therapy for PTSD in Adolescents. *Journal of Clinical Child & Adolescent Psychology*, *46*(4), 500–510. https://doi.org/10.1080/15374416.2015.1012722

MD, P. G. (2020, February 26). *Dopamine fasting: Misunderstanding science spawns a maladaptive fad.* Harvard Health Blog. https://www.health.harvard.edu/blog/dopamine-fasting-misunderstanding-science-spawns-a-maladaptive-fad-2020022618917

Mendell, L. M. (2014). Constructing and deconstructing the gate theory of pain. *Pain*, *155*(2), 210–216. https://doi.org/10.1016/j.pain.2013.12.010

Morse, G. (2006, January 1). *Decisions and Desire*. Harvard Business Review. https://hbr.org/2006/01/decisions-and-desire

National Institute of Mental Health. (2019, December 2). *NIMH» Anxiety Disorders*. Nih.gov. https://www.nimh.nih.gov/health/topics/anxiety-disorders

Newman, M. G., & Llera, S. J. (2011). A novel theory of experiential avoidance in generalized anxiety disorder: A review and synthesis of research supporting a contrast avoidance model of worry. *Clinical Psychology Review*, *31*(3), 371–382. https://doi.org/10.1016/j.cpr.2011.01.008

Oliveira de Carvalho, A., Filho, A. S. S., Murillo-Rodriguez, E., Rocha, N. B., Carta, M. G., & Machado, S. (2018). Physical Exercise For Parkinson's Disease: Clinical And Experimental Evidence. *Clinical Practice & Epidemiology in Mental*

Health, 14(1), 89–98. https://doi.org/10.2174/1745017901814010089

Oscar Berman, M., Blum, K., Chen, T. J., Braverman, E., Waite, R., Downs, W., Arcuri, V., Notaro, A., Palomo, T., & Comings. (2008). Attention-deficit-hyperactivity disorder and reward deficiency syndrome. *Neuropsychiatric Disease and Treatment, 4*(5), 893. https://doi.org/10.2147/ndt.s2627

Poudel, A., & Gautam, S. (2017). Age of onset of substance use and psychosocial problems among individuals with substance use disorders. *BMC Psychiatry, 17*(1). https://doi.org/10.1186/s12888-016-1191-0

Powledge, T. M. (1999). Addiction and the brain. *BioScience, 49*(7), 513–519. https://doi.org/10.2307/1313471

Rogers, S. (2015, June 29). *Constant Expansion; com·mit·ment.* Medium. https://medium.com/@sierrarogers/constant-expansion-com-mit-ment-d51bc7fc7b0

Take Your Pills | Netflix Official Site. (2019, March). Www.netflix.com. https://www.netflix.com/title/80117831

UCL. (2018, November 15). *Uncertainty can cause more stress than inevitable pain.* UCL News.

https://www.ucl.ac.uk/news/2016/mar/uncertainty-can-cause-more-stress-inevitable-pain

Unterwald, E., Eisenstein, T., D'orazio, J., O'gurek, D., Abdallah, R., Rawls, S., & Adler, M. (2017). *PA-SUPPORT Source for Understanding Pain, Prescribing Opioids, and Recovery Treatment Developed by.* https://medicine.temple.edu/sites/medicine/files/files/PA-SUPPORT%20Unterwald%20Temple%20LKSOM%20-R1_0.pdf

Van Zee, A. (2009). The Promotion and Marketing of OxyContin: Commercial Triumph, Public Health Tragedy. *American Journal of Public Health*, 99(2), 221–227. https://doi.org/10.2105/ajph.2007.131714

Whitten, L. A. (2012). Functional Magnetic Resonance Imaging (fMRI): An Invaluable Tool in Translational Neuroscience. In *PubMed*. RTI Press. https://www.ncbi.nlm.nih.gov/books/NBK538909/

Wolff, M., Evens, R., Mertens, L. J., Koslowski, M., Betzler, F., Gründer, G., & Jungaberle, H. (2020). Learning to Let Go: A Cognitive-Behavioral Model of How Psychedelic Therapy

Promotes Acceptance. *Frontiers in Psychiatry, 11.* https://doi.org/10.3389/fpsyt.2020.00005

Printed in Great Britain
by Amazon